The Validation® Training Program

Training Manual
for the Instruction
of Validation

Level 2
The Practice of Validation

**Based on *The Validation Breakthrough*
and other work by Naomi Feil, M.S.W., A.C.S.W.**

**Manual developed by Vicki de Klerk-Rubin, written and edited by
Evelyn Sutton, M.A., and Frances Johnson,
with a grant from The Institute for Quality Improvement
of Long Term Health Care
School of Health Professions
Southwest Texas State University, San Marcos
to the Validation Training Institute, Cleveland, Ohio
Lita Kohn, President, and Naomi Feil, Executive Director**

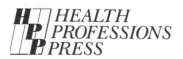

*HEALTH
PROFESSIONS
PRESS*

Baltimore • London • Winnipeg • Sydney

Health Professions Press, Inc.

Post Office Box 10624
Baltimore, Maryland 21285-0624

www.healthpropress.com

Products designed by Four Winds Productions, LLC, Baltimore, Maryland. Manuals typeset by Barton Matheson Willse & Worthington, Baltimore, Maryland, and manufactured in the United States of America by Versa Press, Inc., East Peoria, Illinois. Packaged by the Banta Company, Banta Book Group, Menasha, Wisconsin. Transparencies manufactured by the Banta Company, Menasha, Wisconsin. Videocassettes manufactured by VDO Video, Mt. Airy, Maryland, with sleeves manufactured by Printing Corporation of America, Baltimore, Maryland.

Library of Congress Cataloging-in-Publication Data

Sutton, Evelyn.
    The validation training program : training manual for the instruction of validation : based on "the Validation breakthrough" and other work by Naomi Feil / manual developed and written by Evelyn Sutton.
    2 v. cm.
    The manual is based on both "The Validation breakthrough" and "Validation—the Feil method".
    Includes bibliographical references.
    Contents: level 1. Introduction to validation — level 2. The practice of validation.
    ISBN 1-878812-51-3 (v. 1). — ISBN 1-878812-52-1 (v. 2).
    1. Validation therapy—Handbooks, manuals, etc. 2. Aged—Mental health—Handbooks, manuals, etc. 3. Developmentally disabled aged—Rehabilitation—Study and teaching—Outlines, syllabi, etc. 4. Senile dementia—Patients—Care. 5. Alzheimer's disease—Patients—Care. I. Feil, Naomi. Validation breakthrough. II. Feil, Naomi. V/F validation. III. Title.
RC451.4.A5S88 1999   99-24069
618.97'689—dc21   CIP

Contents

Contributors

Naomi Feil, M.S.W., A.C.S.W., is the Executive Director of the Validation Training Institute, Cleveland, Ohio. She is the creator of Validation, recognized throughout the world as a state-of-the-art intervention for older people with Alzheimer's-type dementia or related disorders. Ms. Feil earned her M.S.W. from Columbia University and studied at the New School for Social Research, Case Western Reserve University, and the University of Michigan. In 1963, she became dissatisfied with traditional therapies for older people with dementia and began to develop her own methods for helping them cope with the disorientation that is sometimes part of the aging process.

Ms. Feil has published numerous books and articles and produced award-winning films and videos on Validation. She is internationally recognized for her work with older people and is one of the most sought-after trainers in the field of aging. More than 7,000 facilities in the United States, Canada, Europe, and Australia have adopted Validation, and more than 70,000 professional and family caregivers have attended her workshops.

Vicki de Klerk-Rubin is the European manager of the Validation Training Institute, a certified Validation trainer, and the coauthor of the 1992 revision of *Validation: The Feil Method.* Ms. Rubin holds a Bachelor of Fine Arts from Boston University and a Master of Business Administration from Fordham University, and is a Dutch-trained registered nurse. Ms. Rubin has given Validation workshops, lectures, and training programs in Austria, Belgium, England, Finland, France, Germany, the Netherlands, and Sweden. She also has worked in numerous nursing facilities in Amsterdam, leading Validation groups and training staff.

Frances Johnson, B.M., M.R.E., earned degrees and certificates from Oklahoma State University, Union Theological Seminary, and the Administrators Training Program at Southwest Texas State University. Her experience with older adults includes work with groups in New York City and Ann Arbor, Michigan, nursing facilities in Texas, and caring for her mother. She has written curricula and articles for the Episcopal Society for Ministry on Aging. She is currently a member of the Eden Alternative Task Force of the Institute for Quality Improvement in Long Term Care at Southwest Texas State University. She assisted in field testing and editing *The Validation Training Program* manuals and has given presentations on the basic principles and techniques of Validation to social workers at Southwest Texas State University, Eden Alternative staff, and family caregivers.

Evelyn Sutton, M.A., is Life Fellow and Adjunct Professor, Institute for Life-Span Development and Gerontology, University of Akron. Ms. Sutton teaches graduate courses in gerontology, with special interests in women's and family issues. Since the early 1980s she has focused on aging and developmental disabilities, conducting training events throughout the United States. Her research has centered on issues of later-life planning, choice, and retirement options for older adults with developmental disabilities. She is the coauthor of numerous articles and several books, including *Older Adults with Developmental Disabilities: Optimizing Choice and Change*, and is the editor of A/DDvantage, an international newsletter on developmental disabilities. Ms. Sutton has been a certified Validation trainer since 1979.

Acknowledgments

The purpose of these training manuals is to extend the pioneering work of Naomi Feil, whose conception and development of Validation as a theory and method of communication with very old disoriented people has contributed immeasurably to the quality of their lives. The manuals are based entirely on her work and in particular on *The Validation Breakthrough*, published in 1993. Her guidance was the essential ingredient in the development of the manuals.

Much credit for the production of these manuals and the development of Validation concepts must be given to Frances Johnson of Austin, Texas. As a former board member of the Institute for Quality Improvement in Long Term Care, she presented, promoted, and promulgated this project. Frances conducted a field test of the document and related videos (*The Four Phases of Resolution* and *Myrna—The Mal-Oriented*). She also led the focus group at which trainees provided helpful feedback on the effectiveness of the manuals as a training instrument.

Vicki de Klerk-Rubin's contributions to the development of the manuals and especially to the exercises used in both Levels 1 and 2 are acknowledged with admiration for her work.

In addition to reviews of the manual drafts by Naomi Feil, other reviewers who provided helpful suggestions for revisions include Lita Kohn, President of the Board of Trustees of the Validation Training Institute; Harvey L. Sterns, Ph.D., Director of the Institute for Life Span Development and Gerontology, University of Akron; Richard Uhle, President of the P.D. Development Corps and President (ret.) of Ohio Presbyterian Homes; and Frances Johnson. Their commitments of time, effort, and expertise are gratefully acknowledged. Validation teacher/trainers Rita O'Brien, Sheila Webster, Mary Ann Anderson, and Colleen Brill are acknowledged for their specific contributions. Many thanks go to Frieda Kramer, whose patience endured throughout multiple revisions to completion of the project.

Finally, appreciation is expressed to the Board of Trustees of the Validation Training Institute for their ongoing support and encouragement and for their dedication to the extension of the principles and techniques of Validation throughout the world.

Evelyn Sutton

The Board of Trustees of the Validation Training Institute is grateful to Southwest Texas State University, Institute for Quality Improvement in Long Term Care, for recognizing, along with us, the need to disseminate information about this valuable and human method. In particular, we wish to recognize Sandy Ransom, Director of the Institute for Quality Improvement in Long Term Care, whose support has been invaluable and unwavering; Frances Johnson, whose energy and enthusiasm made this project possible; Evelyn Sutton, for her intelligence, hard work, and devotion; and Vicki de Klerk-Rubin, to whom goes our deepest gratitude—her energy and constant striving for quality education in Validation worldwide became the guiding force for the Validation training manuals.

Lita Kohn, President, and Naomi Feil, Executive Director, the Validation Training Institute
www.vfvalidation.org

Notes to the Instructor

This training manual provides a standardized curriculum for the introduction of Validation principles, theory, and practice. The manuals are based on the work of Naomi Feil and have been approved by her and the Board of Trustees of the Validation Training Institute. Two books, *Validation: The Feil Method* and *The Validation Breakthrough: Simple Techniques for Communicating with People with "Alzheimer's-Type Dementia,"* are the foundation of the manuals along with other published and unpublished writings and lectures by Feil.

The Validation Training Program was produced with a grant from the Institute for Quality Improvement in Long Term Care, which is affiliated with the School of Health Professions, Southwest Texas State University, San Marcos. It was pilot tested in Texas with a group of health care professionals and practitioners primarily from the Austin-San Marcos area. Researchers at Southwest Texas State University analyzed pre- and posttest results to determine the effectiveness of the manuals as teaching/learning instruments. In addition, the researchers conducted a focus group that comprised two thirds of the pilot class to recommend possible revisions. Naomi Feil observed and rated a random sample of the pilot class in one-to-one practice situations.

Instructor Qualifications

Level 2, "The Practice of Validation," requires experience and an integration of the theory which is acquired only through using Validation with very old disoriented people. Level 2 is taught by certified Validation teachers and trainers who either have received their diplomas from the Validation Training Institute or have been authorized to teach Level 2 by the Validation Training Institute.

How to Use the Level 2 Manual

The Level 2 training manual is to be used by individuals who already possess a large base of knowledge and expertise in Validation. It is a practical guideline for organizing the information on Validation, with specific methods of teaching that information that have proved successful. Many exercises are included within the text so that there is greater focus on practical information than on theory.

Teaching the verbal and nonverbal techniques of Validation can be accomplished in several different ways, but two are essential: 1) each technique must be clearly explained and 2) each technique must be demonstrated clearly and practiced. Handouts that are specific to certain techniques are located at the back of the manual. Overhead transparencies are found in the transparencies folder in the complete *Validation Training Program* kit. Encourage feedback, questions, discussion, role plays, and demonstrations. Teachers and trainers should contribute their own experiences and stories to discussions.

Exercises that illustrate the techniques are included in the text. Often, class members will be asked to divide into groups of two (dyads) to demonstrate the exercises. Role plays and demonstrations are important teaching tools, and the feedback/ criticism and discussion that follows should be constructive. Rather than concentrating on whether what the players are doing is right or wrong, you and the group should focus on what worked well or what might have worked better. During role plays, remind the participants that this is not an acting workshop. Everyone's attention should be on the technique(s) being demonstrated, not on the person(s) playing the role.

Participants in Level 2 training should be trained in Level 1 or its equivalent. Level 2 builds on what was learned and experienced in Level 1. Level 2 includes everything not covered by Level 1 that is necessary to practice individual Validation (with one client at a time). This training manual does not include an examination of group Validation methods and procedures because a group is a complex extension of the one-to-one practice of Validation and requires a different set of skills.

Goals of Level 2: The Practice of Validation

Learners will be able to

- list all verbal and nonverbal Validation techniques
- discuss the techniques that are appropriate to each client
- build a trusting relationship with a very old disoriented person
- demonstrate the use of Validation with a very old disoriented person in each phase of Resolution

Principles of Teaching Adult Learners*

As a trainer, creating a supportive atmosphere in which learners can share experiences and explore new ideas is important to helping them to learn and grow. Listed below are some guidelines for you to help create this atmosphere.

Be open and accepting.   Perhaps the best way to create this feeling is to model it yourself. Point out differences of opinion with the aim of showing the group that these differences are acceptable and that everyone's ideas are valuable and deserve respect.

Remain focused on the task at hand.   The job of keeping participants on task is often difficult; some adult learners go off on tangents that quickly become unrelated to the topic at hand. You are the best judge of when to redirect the group's focus.

Be supportive and flexible.   Keep in mind that there are no wrong answers or feelings, and stress this to the learners. Avoid moralizing and presenting a single "right way" to do things. Encourage learners to discuss what works best for them. You can adjust the lesson plan to meet the needs expressed by the group.

Listen, hear, understand.   A classroom can be the ideal place for adult learners to become aware of good communication skills. You should model empathic listening and understanding. Let learners know that you have really heard what they have said. Focus on what is being said, not on what you are planning to say. Encourage learners to use "I" rather than "we" or "you" in dealing with a very old disoriented person (i.e., do not use phrases such as, "You always hit me when you're upset! What's the matter with you?"). Using "we" or "you" can make the listener feel defensive and tune you out.

Share.   Sharing experiences and feelings with others provides new insights and perspectives on behavior. Perceive the group as a rich resource for learning, and encourage participants to do so as well.

Certification Levels and Requirements

Level 1: Validation Practitioner
Requirements for certification
    Take part in a training course
    Practice individual Validation for at least 6 months
    Show documentation of practical work
    Pass written and practical examinations

---

*Adapted from Adult Resource Center, University of Akron, Akron, Ohio.

Authorizations
  Can practice individual Validation
  Can give short presentations about Validation to small groups
  Can give support to people interested in learning Validation

Abilities
  Empathy
  Exquisitely listen to another human being, hearing the meaning beyond what is spoken
  Can put aside own feelings in order to be nonjudgmental toward the very old disoriented person
  Can observe a very old Maloriented or disoriented person in an organized, careful manner
  Understands the symbols used by very old Maloriented and disoriented adults
  Can diagnose the stage of disorientation (according to Validation theory)
  Can build a warm, trusting relationship with a very old Maloriented or disoriented person
  Can demonstrate all of the Validation principles on a basic level
  Can demonstrate that he or she knows which principles to use with which stage of disorientation
  Can identify basic human emotions and universal needs in very old disoriented people

Knowledge
  Erikson's life stages and tasks, as well as Feil's "Resolution versus Vegetation" stages, and how to apply them to very old disoriented people
  Basic human emotions and universal needs
  Goals of Validation for both the client and the caregiver
  Population for which Validation was developed
  Differences between person with early-onset Alzheimer's disease and a very old disoriented person
  Physical, psychological, and emotional characteristics of the four phases of Resolution
  How Validation differs from and compares with reality orientation, reminiscence, remotivation, and sensory stimulation methods
  Principles of Validation

Level 2: Group Validation Practitioner
Requirements for certification
  Show Level 1 certification (or equivalent) in order to begin this course
  Take part in a training course

Practice group Validation for at least 6 months
Pass written and practical examinations

Authorizations
Can practice group Validation
Can give support to people with Level 1 training and people interested in learning Validation
Can give short presentation about Validation to small groups

Abilities
Perform all of the skills required of a Validation caregiver
Easily recognize the stages of Resolution even when there is blurring of the stages
Form a warm, trusting relationship with a very old Maloriented or disoriented person
Form a Validation group, select group members, assign roles, plan agendas
Work with a Validation team
Share his or her knowledge with others
Select Validation team members
Evaluate the progress of the client
Can demonstrate a successful and correct Validation group
Can demonstrate that he or she has satisfied all of the above

Knowledge
All of the information required of a Validation practitioner
Basic group work theory
Goals of a Validation group
Role of a Validation group leader and that of the co-worker
How to involve other staff members within an institution
Elements of a Validation group

Level 3: Validation Teacher/Trainer
Requirements for certification
Show Level 2 certification in order to begin this course
Demonstrate "didactic" knowledge prior to beginning this course
Take part in a training course
Pass written and practical examinations

Authorizations
Can train people within the context of authorized Validation organizations (AVO) in the following areas: Level 1, Level 2, and family members
Can give information seminars and presentations in cooperation with AVOs

Abilities
    Perform all of the skills required of a Validation practitioner and a group Validation practitioner
    Handle difficult Validation group situations
    Help family members to use Validation with their disoriented relatives
    Teach Validation on Levels 1 and 2
    Give presentations, lectures, and classes in Validation in cooperation with an AVO
    Offer supervision to others in a validating manner
    Explain the theories that are fundamental to Validation: Freud, Jung, Rogers, Piaget, Erikson, Penfield, and neurolinguistic programming
    Work with AVOs

Level 4: Validation Master

Requirements for certification
    Show Level 3 certification
    Experience as a Validation teacher for more than 3 years
    Write an examination work on Validation
    Be authorized by the Validation Training Institute

Authorizations
    Can train, give support and advice to people on Levels 1, 2, and 3 and all people interested in learning Validation
    Can give Validation workshops, seminars, and presentations

Certified Validation Teachers/Trainers

Years of practice with a deep knowledge of Validation principles are essential to an effective implementation of Validation. Individuals who are newly trained and beginning the practice of Validation are urged by the Validation Training Institute (VTI) to contact a certified teacher/trainer for supervision and feedback. Contact VTI for the name of a certified teacher/trainer in your area.

Validation Training Institute
21987 Byron Road East
Shaker Heights, OH 44122
(216) 561-0357
www.vfvalidation.org

The Validation Training Program
Outline for a 1- to 2-Hour Presentation
(General Audiences)

Objectives	Topics	Teaching tools
Define Validation	"Basic Concepts"	Manual 1, topics as indicated
Identify the Resolution struggle	"Validation Defined"	Overhead transparencies "The Four Phases of Resolution"
List the benefits of Validation	"Benefits"	"Goals of Validation"
Identify the goals of the caregiver and the very old disoriented person	"Goals"	Handouts on the physical and psychological characteristics of the four phases of Resolution
Describe the four phases of Resolution	"Characteristics of People in the Four Phases of Resolution"	Video *The Four Phases of Resolution*, plus study guide (see back of manual) *If possible, show the 20-minute video *Communicating with the Alzheimer's-Type Population* (see back of manual for study guide and ordering information)

Outline for In-Service Directors, Home Health
Instructors/Trainers, and Consultants

1-hour sessions for 8 weeks or 2-hour sessions for 4 weeks

Audience:
Nurses and other medical staff, administrators, recreation workers, management, social services workers, maintenance, bookkeeping, housekeeping, dietary staff, home health workers, visiting nurses, occupational and physical therapists, consultants

FIRST HOUR

Objectives	Topics	Teaching tools	Homework
Define Validation	"Basic Concepts"	Manual 1, topics as indicated	Read Introduction to *The Validation Breakthrough*
Identify the Resolution struggle	"Validation Defined"	Overhead transparencies "The Four Phases of Resolution," "Goals," and handouts on the physical and psychological characteristics of the four phases of Resolution	
List the benefits of Validation	"Benefits"		
Describe the four phases of Resolution	"Goals"	Video *The Four Phases of Resolution*, plus study guide (see back of manual), and exercise "Forcing versus Validation"	
Identify the goals of the Validation practitioner	"Characteristics of People in the Four Phases of Resolution"		

SECOND HOUR

Discuss Erikson's stages	Section 2, "Successful Aging," and Section 3, "The Life Stage of Resolution"	Manual 1 topics as indicated; overhead transparencies "Erikson's Life Stages and Life Tasks"; Exercises "Trust Circle," "Rebellion," "Intimacy"; and video *The Seminar Group*, plus study guide (see back of manual)	Read *The Validation Breakthrough*, pp. 10–18
Examine one's unfinished life struggles			
Define integrity and discuss the characteristics of successful aging			

THIRD HOUR

Objectives	Topics	Teaching tools	Homework
List the qualities of a Validation caregiver	Qualities needed by a Validation practitioner	Manual 1, topics as indicated; flip-chart, chalkboard; and exercise "What Does Not Work"	Try to convince a family member, colleague, or friend to change a familiar comfort-able behavior. Does he or she listen?
Define empathy	What is empathy and why is it important in Validation?		
Distinguish empathy from diverting, analyzing, reality orienting, con-fronting, calming, consoling, and redirecting			

FOURTH HOUR

Experience some of the sensory losses that can accom-pany aging	Alzheimer's disease and Validation	Manual 1, topics as indicated; gauze over TV screen, Vaseline on glasses, audiotape of monologue or dialogue; hand-outs on the physical and psy-chological charac-teristics of the four phases of Resolution	
Distinguish the behaviors of a person with early-onset Alzheimer's disease and those of a person with late-onset Alzheimer's disease	Alternative explanations for behavior changes in late life		
Describe the differ-ent benefits of Validation for people with early- or late-onset Alzheimer's disease	Dealing with loss in old age		

FIFTH HOUR

Objectives	Topics	Teaching tools	Homework
Experience "the mind's eye" and "buried awareness"	Basic principles of Validation	Manual 1, topics as indicated	"Buried Awareness"—note a moment when you did not express a painful feeling. How did you feel later? Did you express it later? How did you feel when you did?
List the 12 principles of Validation		Overhead transparencies "12 Principles of Validation," "Erikson's Life Stages" (if necessary), and exercise "Centering"	
Discuss the principle "when painful feelings are expressed and validated, the person feels relief"			

SIXTH HOUR

Objectives	Topics	Teaching tools	Homework
List the physical, psychological, and social characteristics of people who are Maloriented	"Characteristics of People in the Four Phases of Resolution," Phase 1: Malorientation	Manual 1, topics as indicated, *The Validation Breakthrough*, and videos *Myrna—The Mal-Oriented*, plus study guide (see back of manual) and *The Four Phases of Resolution* (first segment)	List male and female authority figures in your workplace and how such figures are used as symbols by Maloriented clients or residents; observe Maloriented clients or residents and attempt to identify what they are trying to express
Describe their body language			
Empathize with people who are Maloriented			

SEVENTH HOUR

Objectives	Topics	Teaching tools	Homework
List the physical, psychological, and social characteristics of people in Time Confusion	"Characteristics of People in the Four Phases of Resolution," Phase 2: Time Confusion	Manual 1, topics as indicated, *The Validation Breakthrough*; exercise "Losing Clock Time"; videos *The Four Phases of Resolution* (second segment) and, if possible, *Communicating with the Alzheimer's-Type Population*	Observe Time Confused clients and residents and attempt to identify what they are trying to express
Empathize with people in Time Confusion			
Describe their body language			

EIGHTH HOUR

Objectives	Topics	Teaching tools	Homework
Describe the physical, psychological, and social characteristics of people in Repetitive Motion and Vegetation	"Characteristics of People in the Four Phases of Resolution," Phases 3 and 4: Repetitive Motion and Vegetation; the use of symbols; "Assessing the Phases of Resolution"; "Summary"	Chalkboard or flipchart; *The Validation Breakthrough*; handouts on the physical and psychological characteristics of the four phases of Resolution; overhead transparencies "Symbols" and "Basic Human Needs"; and exercise "Precise Observation"	
Describe their body language			
Empathize with people in Repetitive Motion and Vegetation			
Understand the use of symbols			

Outline for Family Members of "Alzheimer's-Type" Older Adults
Four 2-Hour Sessions

Audience:

Family home health instructors/trainers, Alzheimer's disease support group directors, social services directors, teaching consultants in home health care, and other professionals working with families and older adults (e.g., clergy, legal guardians)

SESSION ONE

Objectives	Topics	Teaching tools	Homework
Define Validation	"Basic Concepts"	Manual 1, topics as indicated, overhead transparencies "The Four Phases of Resolution" and "Goals," video "The Four Phases of Resolution," and exercise "Forcing versus Validating"	Find out the goals of your "Alzheimer's-type" relative/client/resident, and write down the needs/goals that you can identify
Identify the four phases of Resolution	"Validation Defined"		
Identify the goals of the Validation caregiver	"Benefits"		
Discover the difference (if any) between your goals and those of the Validation caregiver	"Goals"		

SESSION TWO

Objectives	Topics	Teaching tools	Homework
Identify the qualities of the Validation caregiver	Discuss homework from Session One	Manual 1, topics as indicated; chalkboard or flipchart; exercises "What Does Not Work," "Precise Observation," and "Losing Clock Time" (if there is time)	Have at least one 5- to 10-minute listening session with your relative/client/resident, including:
Identify your qualities	Qualities needed in a Validation practitioner		• Listen; do not argue or correct
Discuss empathy; know the difference between empathy and confronting, reality orienting, diverting, calming, arguing, telling the person what to do	What is empathy and why is it important in Validation?		• Listen to his or her voice • Look into his or her eyes • Write down what you hear or see
			Does your relative use you as a symbol for someone from the past? Who?

SESSION THREE

Objectives	Topics	Teaching tools	Homework
Become familiar with the 12 principles of Validation Experience "the mind's eye" Experience "buried awareness"	Discuss homework from Session Two, basic principles of Validation	Manual 1, topics as indicated; overhead transparencies "12 Principles of Validation," "Erikson's Life Stages and Life Tasks"; and exercises "Centering," "Buried Awareness," "Trust Circle" (if there is time), "Rebellion" (if there is time), "Intimacy" (if there is time)	Have at least one 5- to 10-minute listening session with your relative/client/resident, including: • Can you identify any of the Validation principles? • Write down your impressions and feelings

Session Four

Objectives	Topics	Teaching tools	Homework
Know the physical, psychological, and social characteristics of the four phases of Resolution Identify which phase (if any) your relative/client/resident is in	Discuss homework from Session Three, "Characteristics of People in the Four Phases of Resolution," use of symbols, "Assessing the Phases of Resolution," "Summary"	Manual 1, topics as indicated; video *The Four Phases of Resolution* and *Myrna—The Mal-Oriented*; handouts on the physical and psychological characteristics of the four phases of Resolution; overhead transparencies "Symbols" and "Basic Human Needs"; and exercise "Centering" and "Precise Observation"	Use "centering" regularly, listen and look instead of correcting or arguing with relative/client/resident, write down difficult moments

Outline for a 30-Hour, 15-Week Course
Fifteen 2-hour Sessions

Audience:

Participants of all ages, either students or professionals, who wish to learn about Validation

Session	Topics	Teaching tools
1	Give an overview of course, its contents, required text and readings (you may require field work), basic concepts of Validation, qualities needed in a Validation practitioner	Chalkboard or flipchart; video *The Four Phases of Resolution*, plus study guide (see back of manual); overhead transparency "The Four Phases of Resolution"; *The Validation Breakthrough;* and handout "Course Objectives"
2	What empathy is and why it is important in Validation, your attitude toward aging, definition of Validation	Handout "Attitude Toward Aging Scale," exercises "What Does Not Work" and "Forcing versus Validating," and *The Validation Breakthrough*
3	Benefits of Validation, certification information, how Validation was developed	Overhead transparency "Goals," handout "Certification Levels and Requirements," and *The Validation Breakthrough*

Session	Topics	Teaching tools
4	Section 2, "Validation Theory: Successful Aging"	Chalkboard or flipchart; *The Validation Breakthrough*; video *The Seminar Group*, plus study guide (see back of manual)
5	Section 3, "Validation Theory: The Life Stage of Resolution," the life task theory of Erik Erikson, Feil's Resolution stage of life for very old people	Overhead transparency "Erikson's Life Stages and Life Tasks"; exercises "Trust Circle," "Rebellion," "Intimacy"; *The Validation Breakthrough*; video *100 Years to Live*, plus study guide (see back of manual)
6	Section 3, "Validation Theory: The Life Stage of Resolution," the life task theory of Erik Erikson, Feil's Resolution stage of life for very old people	Overhead transparency "Erikson's Life Stages and Life Tasks"; exercises "Trust Circle," "Rebellion," "Intimacy"; *The Validation Breakthrough*; video *100 Years to Live*, plus study guide (see back of manual)
7	The graying of America, who does not need Validation, and diversity is the hallmark of aging	Chalkboard or flipchart and self-supplied materials on "the graying of America"
8	Alzheimer's disease and Validation, alternative explanations for behavior changes in later life, and dealing with losses in old age	Sensitivity-training materials: Vaseline on glasses, TV screen covered with gauze, and tape of monologue
9	Basic principles of Validation	Overhead transparency "12 Principles of Validation"; exercises "Centering," "What Does Not Work," "Buried Awareness"
10	Basic principles of Validation	Overhead transparency "12 Principles of Validation"; exercises "Centering," "What Does Not Work," "Buried Awareness"
11	Characteristics of people in the four phases of Resolution Phase One: Malorientation	Video: *Myrna—The Mal-Oriented*, plus study guide (see back of manual); handouts on the physical and psychological characteristics of people who are Maloriented; *The Validation Breakthrough*

Session	Topics	Teaching tools
12	Phase Two: Time Confusion	Video *The Four Phases of Resolution*, plus study guide (see back of manual); exercise "Losing Clock Time"; *The Validation Breakthrough*
13	Phase Three: Repetitive Motion Phase Four: Vegetation Use of symbols Basic human needs	Chalkboard or flipchart, *The Validation Breakthrough*, overhead transparencies "Symbols" and "Basic Human Needs"
14	Assessing the phase of Resolution, preparation for final assignment	Exercise "Precise Observation" (can also repeat "Centering")
15	Final assignment, Summary	

1 Goals

INSTRUCTOR: In this course you learn how to practice the Validation principles that were discussed in Level 1. The theory of Validation that was explained in the introductory course will be discussed in this course but in another context, the practice of Validation.

I'd like to go back to some topics that were discussed in Level 1: what we can expect from Validation, what results to look for, how to know if you are "doing it right."

(Display the overhead "Positive Effects of Validation.")

You can see from the overhead what your results might be, but results are different from goals. Often, what you try to obtain is not exactly what you get. Sometimes when you try to do something that's very hard, the process gets in the way. So, if my goal is to get a Time Confused woman to stop crying, I can't say to her, "Enough crying now. Be happy." But by using Validation, I might cry with her and talk about what is making her so sad. We could talk about her deepest sadness—remember, we talked about asking the extreme in Level 1? I need to go into the "negative" emotion before reaching a more "positive" reaction.

In the example I just gave, I talked about my goals as a caregiver. What was the "goal" of the Time Confused woman?

(Answers should center on the theme "to express her sadness."
Allow time for one or two answers.)

Often, we are faced with situations in which our caregiver's goals are different from the "goals" of the person we are working with. Both sets of goals are important; however, in Validation we reach our goals by first addressing the goals of the care recipient.

(Display the overhead "Goals of Validation." It is also possible to use the videos *The Four Phases of Resolution* or *Communicating with the Alzheimer's-Type Population.*[1] Allow time to discuss and answer the following questions:

- Which "goals" are expressed by people in Phase 1, and how do they express them?
- Which "goals" are expressed by people in Phase 2, and how do they express them?
- Which "goals" are expressed by people in Phase 3, and how do they express them?)

INSTRUCTOR: Now, the Validation caregiver has different goals.

(Redirect attention to the overhead.
Allow time to discuss and answer the following questions:

- How can we as caregivers express these goals?
- What other goals do we have as caregivers?

Initiate a discussion on "non-Validation goals" such as stopping someone from screaming and shouting when he or she is disrupting others; protecting someone with impaired balance or strength from falling; or not allowing ourselves to be hit or bitten. Try to get people to acknowledge the reality of life in a nursing facility. Recognize that the facility's goals may not coincide with the goals of Validation.)

---

[1]*Communicating with the Alzheimer's-Type Population* is available from Health Professions Press, P.O. Box 10624, Baltimore, MD 21285-0624. Telephone (888) 337-8808. www.healthpropress.com.

2 Determining for Whom Validation is Appropriate

INSTRUCTOR: In the Level 1 course, we said that Validation was not for everyone. Let's get clear about the people for whom Validation is the most appropriate intervention. The reason it's important to be clear is because Validation does not work the same way with all populations. For example, someone with early-onset Alzheimer's disease will not react the same way to Validation as a disoriented older person in Time Confusion. They may exhibit similar behaviors, but you won't get the same results with both people. That can be frustrating and demotivating for caregivers, so I want you to be clear so that your expectations of your work will be more realistic. Let's look at the characteristics that Feil has identified to define what is a very old disoriented person.

(Show the overhead "Goals of a Very Old Disoriented Person," and
read each description. Allow brief time for discussion.)

INSTRUCTOR: What illnesses cause disorientation in older people?

(Allow a few minutes for participants to come up with their own ideas
[examples: Parkinson's disease, Korsakoff's syndrome, multi-infarct
dementia, psychosis]. You also could discuss the differences between
someone with apraxia or aphasia and a disoriented person.)

INSTRUCTOR: The key differences between someone who is disoriented because of a physical illness or a purely psychiatric problem such as psychosis and a very old disoriented person are

1. A very old disoriented person's disorientation comes from a combination of physical, psychological, and social losses. This combination always builds up over time.

2. A very old disoriented person's confusion has a purpose: to resolve unfinished business from the past and/or to escape the unbearable reality of the present.

(Allow time to discuss these differences. If there is enough time, show the video *100 Years to Live* or *The Seminar Group*, which show the differences between oriented and disoriented older people. Ask participants to identify the factors that lead to disorientation. Use the study guides included at the back of this manual to prompt you.)

INSTRUCTOR: Remember that Validation is appropriate for people who

- are 80 years old and older
- are resolving unfinished issues from their past, are trying to escape present reality because it's so unpleasant, or are expressing their basic human needs and therefore live in their own version of reality
- are unable to accept the losses associated with aging

Validation works best with people whose disorientation comes from physical *and* psychological factors.

3 Verbal and Nonverbal Validation Techniques

INSTRUCTOR: How do you communicate with a Maloriented or disoriented older person using Validation? What do you say? How do you say it? Do you use a loud or a soft tonc of voice? You need to be very sure that you understand the theory of Validation before you begin to use the techniques. It is crucial that you are able to identify what phase of Resolution the older person is in because some of these techniques are appropriate only for a particular phase. Once you've identified the phase, you can use certain Validation techniques to communicate with the person. Feil has laid out 15 verbal and nonverbal techniques and the phases for which they're appropriate.

(Distribute handout and display overhead "Phases of Resolution and Their Appropriate Validation Techniques.")

INSTRUCTOR: The first is "centering."

Centering

INSTRUCTOR: As a Validation worker, you must put aside your own emotions and any lingering thoughts before communicating seriously with an older person who is Maloriented or disoriented. You're trying to build empathy with the older person, and self-absorption just gets in the way. So you need to calm yourself, put your stress behind you, and put away your own feelings for awhile. Have you ever felt that you couldn't concentrate on what someone was saying because you were preoccupied with your own feelings? You need to clear your own mind and emotions in order to be open to another human being. There are lots of different ways of clearing yourself of distracting feelings and thoughts. How many of you meditate? Do yoga or stress-management exercises? What about relaxation exercises?

(Allow time for a few responses.)

INSTRUCTOR: All of those are good ways of clearing your mind and your heart so that you can step into the shoes of another human being. Feil talks about "centering." Centering is a way of focusing your energy and thoughts on finding balance within yourself. In the process of centering, distracting emotions and thoughts are put aside so that you can concentrate on the important work of Validation.

(If time permits, do the centering exercise on
p. 55 of the Level 1 manual. This is recommended in
place of the brief version described below.)

INSTRUCTOR: Let's try centering as a group. First, close your eyes. Now, take your hand and place it on your lower abdomen. Concentrate all of your thoughts on that spot and begin to take slow, deep breaths, in through your nose and out through your mouth. Take eight slow, deep breaths. Concentrate only on breathing. Put away all of your other thoughts, all of your inner dialogue, and breathe.

(Allow 1–2 minutes for participants to settle into their breathing.)

INSTRUCTOR: Do you feel more relaxed? Calm? Once you do, you are centered. When you are centered, you can focus on the older person who is Maloriented or Time Confused and begin to find empathy for him or her. Validation takes a lot of energy, and it takes your full attention. Centering will help you to find the energy and achieve the proper frame of mind. You must center before you do anything else, even before you move toward the person you're going to communicate with. Let's try centering one more time.

(Repeat the brief version of the centering exercise.)

INSTRUCTOR: Let's see how important centering is when you are actually practicing Validation.

(Start the video *Myrna—the Mal-Oriented* at
the point after which Myrna has fallen, when the Validation
caregiver is trying to make contact with her. When the video ends,
allow time for a discussion of how centering helped the Validation
caregiver, what impressed participants the most about how the
Validation caregiver used the techniques, what they didn't like, what
seemed difficult, and what seemed easy.)

INSTRUCTOR: Let's review several verbal techniques that work with people in Maloriention or Time Confusion. They don't really work in the later phases of Resolution: People in the Repetitive Motion phase usually don't respond to these verbal approaches, and, of course, the approaches wouldn't be appropriate for anyone in Vegetation. We're going to look at "asking factual questions," "rephrasing," "asking the extreme (polarity)," "imagining the opposite," "reminiscing," and "identifying and using the preferred sense."

Asking Factual Questions

INSTRUCTOR: The second Validation technique is asking factual questions. Because you know that Maloriented people are afraid of feelings, ask them for the facts about anything that seems to be occupying their thoughts and attention. What questions can you ask to help you get the facts? Very specific questions: Who? What? When? Where? *However, a Validation caregiver never asks why.* Maloriented people do not want insight. They don't want to think about why, much less tell you about it. The Maloriented person says to you, "Someone is stealing my jewelry." So, you ask, "*What* is it that's missing? *Who* do you think might have stolen it? *When* did you first notice it was gone? Is it the jewelry you keep in the blue velvet case or the jewelry you keep in your drawer?" Ask very specific questions, and you will probably get very specific answers. Find a gentle way to con-

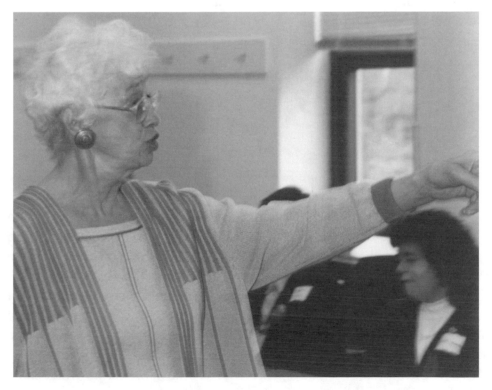

Naomi Feil demonstrates the verbal technique "asking factual questions" during a Validation workshop.

clude the conversation, and it will end in all probability with the woman's feeling better, maybe even forgetting about the "robbery." These fact-finding questions will build trust with the very old Maloriented person. The questions don't suggest that you don't believe her. They aren't intended to distract her, and they're not threatening to her in any way. They tell her that you're taking her complaint seriously and that you know how it feels when something precious is lost. You don't argue with her if she blames others. You don't confront her with your own set of facts. You accept what she is saying because you know there's a reason behind the behavior. Deep down, on a hidden level of awareness, the Maloriented woman knows that she has hidden her jewelry, but she doesn't want to bring the knowledge into consciousness. This is a perfect example of the basic Validation principle that we talked about in Level 1: All of us have many levels of awareness. The Maloriented woman feels robbed because she's experienced many losses, and she hasn't coped well with them. She's an unhappy person. She needs to blame someone so that she can feel better. She may feel that she's losing her identity, her independence, her usefulness. What she's upset about probably is not her jewelry, but it is a real feeling of being robbed.

Let's spend a few minutes role-playing asking factual questions. Everyone find a partner, and decide which of you will play "A" and which will play "B." "A" will be a person with a problem—let's say a book she's been reading is "missing." "B" can ask the factual questions that will explore the situation.

> (Allow about 5 minutes for the role play and
> then ask for brief feedback after the activity.)

Rephrasing

INSTRUCTOR: The third technique is rephrasing. Rephrasing is more than active listening; it builds trust because you show by your tone of voice as well as by your words that you believe the feelings the person has. You repeat what the person has said in your own words, using all of your energy to pick up the rhythm of the older person's speech and his or her tone of voice. You speak with an emotion that matches the emotion that the very old person is expressing. This is empathy in action. You don't diffuse or redirect what you hear. Instead, you help the older person to fully express her feelings. If a very old woman says, "I want to die," you respond by picking up the woman's pitch and tone of voice. The woman's voice was low and the tempo slow. You ask, slowly, in a low voice, "You mean you don't want to live anymore?" The old woman may then share with you how life is, now that she can't see. She expresses her despair to you fully and freely, and she feels better. She has been heard. Someone has listened to her with empathy, not tried to make her think of other things and forget her troubles. The old woman recognizes that this person (you), whoever she is, believed her when she said she wanted to die. Rephrasing directly addresses the psychological principle that feelings lose their strength when they are expressed. Let's try a rephrasing exercise.

(Introduce the exercise "Rephrasing." Ask participants to select a partner to work with, and decide who will be "A" and who will be "B." Allow time for feedback and then ask participants to switch roles.)

Asking the Extreme (Polarity)

INSTRUCTOR: The fourth Validation technique is polarity, or asking the extreme. This technique is very effective with Maloriented people. When you ask the extreme, you ask, What was the worst? What was the best? What was the most? What was the least? You listen with empathy. You know that Maloriented people need to express their emotions, but they can't say in a direct way how they feel. Asking the extreme helps people who are Maloriented tell you more. You would never use an

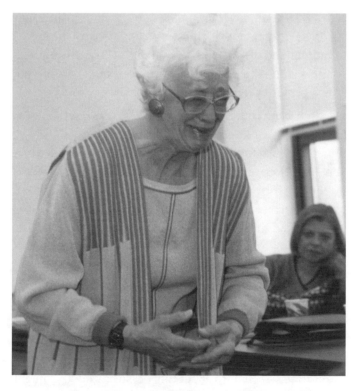

Naomi Feil role-plays an 87-year-old woman who is telling the story of the loss of her first child after being asked the extreme—"What was the worst?"—by a validating caregiver.

Exercise: Rephrasing

Purpose—To experience relief and lessening of anxiety when one is vali-dated, and to build trust with a very old disoriented person.

Instructions

"A" and "B" face one another. "A" takes a moment to center. *Instructor to "A":* Close your eyes and think of someone who annoys you. Can you picture this person? The color of the eyes? The hair? What is the person wearing? Can you see the person walk into the room? Does the person walk fast? Slow? How does the person sit? Now, the person is beginning to talk. How does the person talk—Fast? Slow? Whiney? How do you feel when you are with this person? Does your heart beat faster? Do your muscles tense up? Do you want to walk away? Punch the person? Do you get a headache? Is there a familiar smell to this person? A certain body odor or perfume? See, hear, and feel the person's presence.

"A" opens his or her eyes. *Instructor to "A":* Find something in "B" that reminds you of this annoying person. Tell "B" what you don't like about him or her. (If you can't find anything in "B" that reminds you of this person, tell "B" about him or her.)

Instructor to "B": You know that "A" is using you as a substitute for someone else. Even so, you might feel hurt. Try now to put away the hurt. You know that "A" is not talking about *you.* You know that "A" needs to release some long-stifled emotions, and stifled emotions produce pain. Before you can rephrase, "B," you must center to free yourself of your own emotions.

"B" spends time centering. *Instructor to "B":* Look at "A's" lower lip. Is it tight? Tighten your own lower lip. "B," listen closely to "A's" voice. Is it high or low pitched? Is it monotone? Does the inflection of the voice go up at the end of a sentence? Repeat what "A" has said in your own words, but don't say it in a flat tone of voice. Pick up the pitch and tempo of "A's" voice, but don't mimic "A". When you rephrase and pick up the person's rhythms, the very old Maloriented or disoriented person knows that you are really listening and that you care. The person begins to talk more and trusts you more.

(*Note:* You can only rephrase once or twice. Otherwise, the old person will ask, "Are you deaf?" Rephrasing takes energy, not time.)

(Give everyone a chance to practice rephrasing a few times.)

Instructor to group: So, how did it go? Did "A" feel that "B" was really listening? Did "A" want to tell "B" more about this person? Did "A" begin to trust "B"?

analytical approach and say, "Let's sit down and talk. You seem to be angry or sad about something." People who are Maloriented do not come to you for counseling; they don't want to get in touch with their feelings. People who are Maloriented have denied their feelings for seven or eight decades, so they probably won't open up now. By using polarity you stick to the facts—the worst, the best, the most, the least. Feelings come out *indirectly.* Maloriented people feel better when they are listened to. Someone who cares is asking them to tell more. For example, a Maloriented old man says, "I *will not* take a bath! The water isn't clean!" The validating caregiver knows that there is meaning behind his words, a real reason for his attitude toward bathing. Maybe he is having a flashback to a time when he nearly drowned or was threatened by a flood. Using polarity, you ask, "What is the worst thing that can happen if you take a bath?" "I might fall and hurt myself," he answers. You ask, "What can you do to stop yourself from falling?" Often, the person who is Maloriented comes up with a solution that calms the situation, however, he may not want to get in touch with his fear of drowning or any other feeling he may have about water. The Validation caregiver is not going to "fix" the very old Maloriented person or make that person change his ways.

Imagining the Opposite

INSTRUCTOR: The fifth technique is imagining the opposite, the opposite of the situation that the person is complaining about, the opposite of the situation that's causing anxiety. For instance, a Maloriented woman insists that there is a man under her bed:

Validation caregiver: Is he always there? Is there any time when he is not there?
Maloriented woman: When I'm with someone, not just by myself, he's never there.
Validation caregiver: Was someone always with you when you were younger?
Maloriented woman: Oh, my husband never left my side!
Validation caregiver: Never?
Maloriented woman: Well, he was in the Army for 3 years, and I was alone.
Validation caregiver: How did you cope with being alone?
Maloriented woman: Oh, I looked at my husband's pictures and listened to our favorite records.

You can see that imagining the opposite can lead you into another Validation technique, reminiscing. What might the Validation caregiver do or say then?

(Let the group respond and come up with the
answer: She helps the older woman find pictures of
her husband and recordings of their favorite songs.)

Exercise: Imagining the Opposite and Reminiscing

Purpose—practice verbal Validation techniques; imagining the opposite and reminiscing can sometimes lead to a lessening of the behavior problem if the older person can call on a familiar coping method.

Instructions

"A" and "B" face one another.

Instructor to "A": Center yourself while I lead "B" in imagining a difficult situation.

Instructor to "B": Center yourself and remember a difficult situation that occurred recently. You might have lost your keys, your child was sick and you had to go to work, you had a fight with your husband or wife—whatever feels strongest to you right now. Can you see the situation in your mind's eye? Who is there? What are you wearing? What do you hear? Is there music, a voice, silence? What do you feel? Is it hot or cold? Is your heart pounding? Try to experience the situation now.

Instructor to "A": Observe your partner's face, shoulders, breathing, and posture. Match the energy that you sense coming from "B."

Instructor to "B": Open your eyes [*if they were closed*] and briefly tell "A" about the difficult situation that you were in.

Instructor to "A": Ask your partner to imagine the opposite. Ask your partner, "Has this happened to you before? What happened? How did you handle it then?"

INSTRUCTOR: Imagining the opposite and the sixth Validation technique, reminiscing, helped the Maloriented woman in the example find a familiar (to her) way to survive stress. Here's another example: A very old man living in a nursing facility is Maloriented.

Man: They are poisoning my food!
Validation practitioner: Is there any time that they don't poison your food?
Man: When my daughter visits me and eats at my table. They don't dare poison the food when she's there.

If the Validation caregiver builds trust and becomes a daughter-substitute, then the Maloriented man won't spend as much time accusing others of poisoning his food. He can feel safe with the trusted Validation caregiver.

Let's try some of the verbal techniques we've been learning about. Get into your dyads.

(Give participants enough time to respond between
each instruction of the exercises.)

INSTRUCTOR: There's no doubt about it—imagining the opposite, asking the extreme, or even asking the who, what, when and where questions—they all take imagination. That means thinking on your feet, being creative. In the beginning you'll worry about choosing the right technique for the right situation or wanting to keep the conversation going and bring it to a positive end. Pauses may feel endless, or you may be in too much of a hurry. Relax. Center yourself. Focus on the person you are working with. You need to be very aware of that person. Concentrate. Put yourself in his shoes. Use empathy. Once you can see through the eyes of the person you are talking to, the questions will come naturally.

Don't worry about making mistakes. Even if you ask the wrong questions the Maloriented or disoriented person will forgive you IF you have built a trusting relationship and you are honest. The wise older person knows that you mean well when you ask questions out of interest and caring. If you are asking questions just to ask questions, then the wise old person will most likely ignore you, get angry, or fall asleep. Remember, the first step in Validation is empathy. Once you demonstrate empathy, the techniques will work. Without empathy, all of the techniques that you learn in this course will not help you make contact and communicate with your client.

Validation takes focus and energy, not necessarily clock time. Feil suggests that validating someone for 5 minutes, three times a day is often enough, but the frequency will vary with the situation and the person you are validating. A Maloriented person can concentrate longer than a person in Repetitive Motion. A person in Vegetation needs only the length of time it takes to sing an old, familiar song.

Reminiscing

INSTRUCTOR: Reminiscence is technique number 6. We've talked a little about reminiscence and practiced it. The technique is easy, effective, and can be enjoyable, for both the older adult and you. For older people, reminiscing is natural and age-appropriate. The trust that has been built between you keeps growing because you are genuinely interested in what is being told to you about the person's past. You want to know as much about this person as you can, and what he or she tells you about the past can tell you much.

Reminiscing can be used with people who are Maloriented or Time Confused. It can help solve a problem, as it did for the lonely woman who believed that there was a man hiding under her bed. People in these phases of Resolution are thinking a lot about the past, sometimes trying to solve a lingering problem or tie up loose ends. Not everyone reminisces happily, however. Some people are absorbed by the misery in their past and just want someone to listen to how they feel about it. You need to be able to tune into the bad memories as well as the good if you're going to be an effective Validation caregiver.

Identifying and Using the Preferred Sense

INSTRUCTOR: Validation technique 7—identifying and using the preferred sense—is a bit of a challenge as well. Assuming that a person doesn't have a sensory impairment, everyone uses the five senses. As babies we are bombarded with sensations. We are just learning to take everything in. Neurolinguistic programming theory says that as babies each of us chooses one sense to be the primary sense. It is through that sense that we first take in information from our environment. Some babies choose the auditory sense—those babies respond first to sounds, other babies are kinesthetic. Those babies respond most willingly to touch and feelings, whereas the majority of babies choose the visual sense—they use their eyes first and then respond with their other senses.

INSTRUCTOR: How does identifying a person's preferred sense help us to communicate with very old disoriented people? What good does it do? It makes communication easier, and it builds trust. You are speaking the other person's language when you match your words to the person's preferred sense. If the old person uses "seeing" words, the validating caregiver builds trust by also using "seeing" words. For example, when a Maloriented person says, "I see a man under the bed," the caregiver asks, "What does he look like? What is he wearing?

Exercise: Identifying Our Preferred Sense

Instructions

"A" and "B" sit at a comfortable distance facing one another.

Instructor to "A" : Center and then think of a happy time that you've had in the past 2 or 3 weeks.

Instructor to "B" : I want you to carefully observe "A." Listen to what "A" says and pick out the first sensory verb that "A" uses (for example, "hearing," "seeing," "feeling," "smelling," "tasting.") This sensory verb most likely describes "A's" preferred sense.

Instructor to "A" : Picture yourself in that happy place or at that happy event. What time of day was it? Was it dark or light? Were you inside or outside? What was around you? What were you wearing? Who were you with? What were they wearing? Were you sitting? Standing? What sounds did you hear? Was it loud? Noisy? How did you feel? Did your heart beat fast with excitement? Did your muscles feel relaxed? Open your eyes and tell "B" about your happy experience.

After "B" has identified "A's" preferred sense, they should switch roles and repeat the exercise.

Discussion

Could each person identify his or her preferred sense? Allow sufficient time for discussion.

(Take a few minutes to make sure each participant understands the
technique of using the preferred sense, and why it is used in
Validation. Clarify the meaning if necessary.)

INSTRUCTOR: How do you find out which sense the person prefers? The best way
is to do it by observing and listening. Ask yourself questions: How does he use his
eyes, ears, or hands? Does she notice color, form, or sounds? When he speaks does
he use words like *look* and *see* or descriptive words that tell you that he uses his
eyes a lot? Does she use words or phrases like *I hear* or *it sounds like,* or words
that describe sounds, words like *loud* and *soft*? Does this person respond better to
music or to a colorful bouquet of flowers? If the person is verbal, you can sometimes ask him or her to tell you something that happened in the past. Then, as in
the exercise, you can pick up on the first word he or she uses that refers to one of
the senses. It's more detective work, of course, but it can pay off if you identify the
preferred sense and then use words and phrases that reflect or appeal to that sense.
Here's a list of words that relate to each of the senses.

(Distribute the handout
"Words that Relate to a Person's Preferred Sense.")

INSTRUCTOR: You can practice this technique with family or friends until you become really sharp at identifying the preferred sense. Then, in conversation, practice using words that appeal to that sense.

Maintaining Eye Contact and a Caring Tone of Voice

INSTRUCTOR: Techniques 8 and 9 are quite simple nonverbal Validation techniques—maintaining genuine, close eye contact and using a low, clear, caring tone
of voice. You may already be using these techniques in your work with older people because for many caregivers, they just come naturally. We need to be aware,
however, of when and with whom it is appropriate to use direct eye contact. Eye
contact stimulates energy in people in Phases Two and Three, must be used with
care for individuals in Phase One, and is a goal for people in Phase Four. People
who are Time Confused, in particular, feel more secure with direct eye contact. If
they've been wandering around, possibly searching for a loved one, eye contact
often reduces the anxiety they feel. The validating caregiver projects genuine care
and concern through the eyes, and the Time Confused person sees that. The caregiver becomes, for the moment, the thing that anchors them.

Maintaining close or direct eye contact is not necessarily good for individuals who are Maloriented because they often feel threatened by it. They need psy-

chological space and respectful distance, so be sensitive to their need. Caregivers often receive eye contact from individuals in Phase Four as a result of validating them. Here, making direct eye contact becomes a goal.

Using a low, clear, caring tone of voice sounds simple enough, but we don't always hear ourselves and realize how we sound to others, and we don't recognize the effect our tone of voice has on those around us. Listen to yourself as you give care. A harsh tone of voice can cause a person to become agitated or angry. Such a voice could trigger memories of punishment or disapproval with disoriented individuals. Listen to yourself for the "parent voice," that instructive, almost condescending tone that parents use when correcting their children's behavior. Remember that the disoriented older adult is not a child and responds like an adult to respect when it's offered. Show respect for him or her with your voice. A clear, caring tone of voice carries a positive message and can trigger warm and nurturing memories. Don't all of us respond positively to those tones of voice? The tone of voice you use makes the difference between affirmation and doubt, respect and tolerance, and very old people *can* tell the difference. Let's spend a few minutes role-playing different tones of voice.

(After the volunteers practice different tones of voice,
let the others give feedback: For example, "Your tone of
voice made me think of . . . " or "I felt _____ when you said that.")

INSTRUCTOR: Now we're going to learn about several techniques that are appropriate and helpful for people in Time Confusion and Repetitive Motion. You probably won't use them with people who are Maloriented because they do not want to be touched and their language skills are still intact.

Using Four Basic Human Emotions

INSTRUCTOR: Very old disoriented people no longer communicate solely on a verbal level. Because the brain's centers of logical thinking and speech have deteriorated, they turn increasingly to emotions and movements to express human needs. Therefore the validating caregiver must communicate on an emotional level to enter their world. There are four basic human emotions—love, hate, fear, and sadness—and each basic emotion has many levels of intensity—joy, happiness, fury, anger, panic, worry, guilt, despair, grief, and so on. Like all human beings, the validating caregiver has experienced all of these emotions and can accept them. By using careful observation techniques we can recognize the signs and characteristics of these emotions in others. Sometimes the signs and characteristics are obvious; sometimes they are subtle. Remember to put away your own emotions and center, or you can't validate another person. You don't want to be too busy with your own emotions and run the risk of projecting your feelings onto the client.

Expressing the Emotion with Emotion

INSTRUCTOR: Let's move on to number 10. The Validation caregiver listens for the emotion being expressed by the very old disoriented person and discerns what it is. Pick up on the emotion. Express the emotion with emotion—match his or her tone. The very old person is liable to trust you if your tone of voice matches his or hers. That is empathy, the cornerstone of Validation. For instance, an old gentleman in Phase Three shakes his cane and shouts, "You susfpatches. Set the sofadrakene out! Damnit!" The Validating caregiver picks up on his anger and says in a voice that matches his intensity, "Mr. Poncello, did *they* do *that* to you?" In the example, using ambiguity ("they" and "that") and expressing the emotion with emotion are combined. The old man knows that someone really is listening, so he opens his eyes. Once eye contact between the caregiver and Mr. Poncello is established, Validation can begin. The caregiver asks, "How many of them were there? Two or three?" Mr. Poncello nods his head and his voice gets a little softer as they talk. The validating caregiver may never find out what happened to him, but the communication continues. Mr. Poncello is no longer alone with his anger. He has been heard and validated. Let's practice expressing the emotion with emotion. (See exercise on p. 35.)

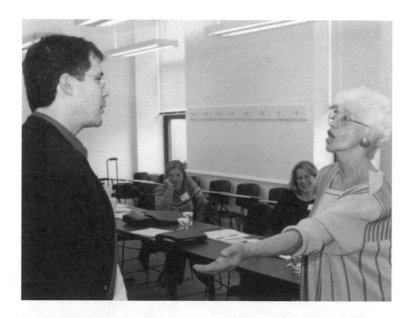

Expressing the emotion with emotion is demonstrated as Naomi Feil asks the older man being role-played by a Validation training participant how many "susfpatches" there were.

Exercise: Expressing the Emotion with Emotion

Purpose—To practice using nonverbal Validation

Instructions

Pair up into groups of two, and decide who will be "A" and who will be "B." Sit relatively close, facing one another. Leave enough room between you and the next dyad so that you feel you have some privacy. Take a few moments to center yourselves.

Instructor to "A": Close your eyes and think of someone you love. Picture the color of their eyes, their hair. What are they wearing? Can you see the person walk into the room? Does the person walk fast or slow? How does the person sit—do they plunk into the chair? Cross their legs? Now, picture the person you love beginning to talk. How do they sound? How do you feel when you are with this person? Does your heart beat faster? Do your muscles tense up? Do you want to walk away? Kiss them? Keep your eyes closed while I talk to "B."

Instructor to "B": Look at "A's" face. Look at the lips, the chin, the cheeks, the neck. Notice "A's" body language, the way "A" is sitting. Look at "A's" hands. Notice the way "A" is breathing. Can you feel a change in "A's" energy? Try to notice everything in order to pick up the emotion that you believe "A" is feeling. Now, think of a situation where you felt the same way. Tell "B" the emotion that both you and "A" are feeling, and say it using that emotion.

Instructor to "A": If "B" is correct and has matched your emotion, open your eyes. This is the beginning of your relationship. If "B" has not matched your emotion, keep your eyes closed because "B" needs to observe more carefully and try again.

Feedback

When everyone has finished the exercise, lead a discussion about what happened. What clues told you what your partner was feeling? "A," when your partner's voice matched what you were feeling, how did that make you feel?

Switch roles.

Using Ambiguity

INSTRUCTOR: Technique 11 is ambiguity, which means using pronouns like "he," "she," "someone," "it," or "they"; numbers; or prepositions like "up," "down," "in," or "out" to fill in during conversation when the person doesn't seem to make sense. You'll find that very old disoriented people, especially those in Phase Three, often move the tongue, lips, or teeth and create new sounds because they've lost the dictionary words. He uses sounds and facial movements instead of speech to communicate. Don't worry about correcting the person's speech. Try helping him or her communicate by filling in what is needed in order to make contact.

When physical deterioration in the brain limits or destroys speech, very old disoriented people return to early-learned, permanently stored memories. They go back to movements acquired before they learned to talk—movements of the tongue, teeth, lips, and jaw. To communicate with them, Validation practitioners use vague, ambiguous pronouns, numbers, and prepositions to substitute for dictionary words. Validating caregivers are able to communicate without understanding the meaning of their unique word combinations. For example, an old woman smiles and sees with her mind's eye: "The tifles of the spoofles fell and we schwitzled there." The validating caregiver observes that the old woman is feeling joy and says, "You loved that. Were there two or three?" "That" and the numbers "two or three" are vague, allowing the woman to choose the correct answer. If the caregiver had asked her, "How many were there?" she couldn't reply because she couldn't think of the dictionary words. The practitioner must supply the words, and the old person will pick up the one that fits.

Let's do an exercise that uses ambiguity. (See exercise on p. 37.)

Mirroring

INSTRUCTOR: Number 12 is another nonverbal technique called mirroring. Mirroring means that you try to match the action and the emotion of the person you want to communicate with. You observe whatever movement the person is making—rocking, tapping, swaying, or folding the arms—and then match it. If you're successful, you grow closer to the person, more in touch with his or her world.

You may not be comfortable using this mirroring technique in its most overt way with some clients. For example, people in Time Confusion and Repetitive Motion are typically free and uninhibited in their movements. Sometimes it's not easy for professional caregivers to let themselves go and do things like pound on a table or rock back and forth. It's understandable. They have many other roles to play. In

Exercise: Using Ambiguity

Purpose—To practice communicating with individuals in Phase 2, Time Confusion, and Phase 3, Repetitive Motion, who are losing speech and can no longer communicate using dictionary words

Instructions

Pair up into groups of two. Decide who is "A" and who is "B." Sit facing one another and center.

Instructor to "A": Repeat a familiar saying, nursery rhyme, or prayer to "B" quickly, so that the sounds blur and "B" can hardly understand the words. As you speak, feel a strong emotion, for instance, anger, love, fear, or sadness.

Instructor to "B": Listen to "A's" tone of voice. Carefully observe "A" from eyes to feet, probing for emotions as "A" speaks. Once you feel you've figured out "A's" emotion, express it in the same emotion by using a vague pronoun, number, or preposition. Communicate in this manner for 3 minutes.

Example

"A" (with anger, low voice, arched eyebrows, eyes and lips tight, hands making fists): PeterPiperpickedapeckofpickledpeppers.

"B" (matching "A's" anger): Did that make your angry?   "A" answers.
"B": Did they hurt you?   "A" answers.
"B": Were you inside or outside?   "A" answers.
"B": Were there two or three?   "A" answers.
"B": Did they leave you alone?   "A" answers.

"A" answers using unique word combinations such as "Yes, Peterpuppostems."

"B" listens again, looks at "A," and expresses "A's" emotion using ambiguous pronouns, prepositions, and numbers.

At the end of 3 minutes, reverse roles.

Feedback

Another way for participants to practice ambiguity is to show the video *The Four Phases of Resolution.* Cue it up to the part where Janet says, "But that is why I said . . .," and stop the tape. Encourage students to come up with possible responses. Discuss what might work and what might be irritating.

such instances, you can mirror more subtly by mirroring someone's facial expression or breathing. You can mirror the way someone walks. You can speak with the same tone of voice. You can match the step of the person as you walk with him or her. (See exercise on p. 39.)

Linking Behavior with an Unmet Human Need

INSTRUCTOR: The 13th technique is linking the person's behavior with an unmet human need. What human needs do people in later life have?

(Show overhead "Basic Human Needs."
Facilitate a brief discussion around how we express those needs in our own lives. When the discussion ends, return the Validation techniques overhead to the projector.)

INSTRUCTOR: Throughout life all of us need to love and be loved. Love is a very basic human need and it doesn't evaporate just because we get to be 80 or 90 years old. Human beings also need to feel needed, to feel useful. Sitting in a chair hour after hour would certainly make anyone feel extremely useless. Sometimes the human need is expressed in repetitive movements that represent work. For example, very old disoriented people may pound repeatedly on a table or a woman may file things in her purse over and over again. When speech fails, familiar movements take its place. People who have worked all of their lives remember the rhythm of

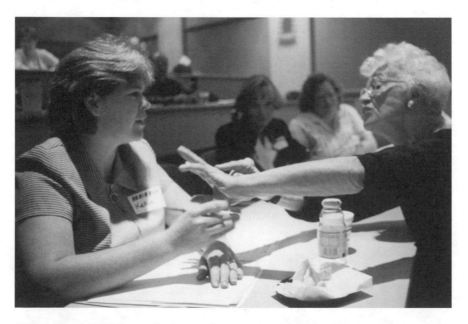

"Often, people use symbols or whatever is at hand to try to express their emotion or their need."

Exercise: Mirroring Movement

Purpose—To practice the nonverbal Validation technique, mirroring

Very old disoriented people, who move to inner rhythms, will communicate when someone genuinely mirrors their movements. The validating caregiver follows the old person's lead.

Instructions

Pair up into groups of two. Decide who will be "A" and who will be "B." You can either sit or stand to do the exercise. Face one another and take time to center. Do not speak during the exercise.

Instructor to "A": Choose a simple task to do, like brushing your hair, brushing your teeth, shaving, putting on make-up, whatever you like.

Instructor turns to "B."

Instructor to "B": Watch "A" carefully as the task is performed. I want you to match "A's" movements exactly—match the rhythms, pick up the same breathing, and so forth. Go slowly.

Instructor to both: When you have become one, I'd like "B" to initiate another movement, and "A" should mirror "B."

Participants should alternate mirroring one another's movements, and should not tell their partner when they are going to initiate the new movement.

their work and feel comfortable with the movements involved. Remember how Mrs. Dorsey mimed sewing in the video *100 Years to Live*? She had been a seamstress during her working life. The motions involved in sewing were familiar and comfortable to her.

People need to express their feelings. Some of us can do that easily and others can say how they feel only under very special conditions. Strong feelings connected with major life events and crises that are not expressed do not go away; they remain in the subconscious and, many times, come back years later. Remember the Validation principle—feelings that are expressed are relieved.

Often, people use symbols or whatever is at hand to try to express their emotion or their need. As you carefully observe your client, ask yourself what human need these symbols or motions represent to him or her. Many very old people need to express deep emotions. We *all* need someone to listen to us and to share our mood, whatever it happens to be. The validating caregiver is there to listen with empathy, to catch the person's mood and help relieve the tension that has built up because emotions have been bottled up. Do you think you can do that? This technique isn't the easiest, and it really depends almost entirely on your observation and listening skills. Let's do an exercise that demonstrates how you can link a client's behavior with an unmet human need. Get back into pairs. (See exercise on p. 41.)

Touching

INSTRUCTOR: Touching is a technique that you might expect to use in Validation, but it's not for general use. Maloriented people usually don't appreciate touching. They avoid it. They want to preserve their psychological space. They want to protect themselves from intimacy or from expressing feelings. People who are Time Confused welcome human touch. They've lost a lot of their inhibitions, and sometimes they're in a kind of haze, where the world seems dim and unfamiliar. (Remember, we're talking about very old people who have vision and hearing losses.) For the most part, Time Confused people have lost track of time and place. Often, they don't recognize people and confuse them with people from the past. It is possible, however, to move into their world.

People in Repetitive Motion have withdrawn even more deeply into their own world than have Time Confused people. They're only vaguely, if at all, aware of the world around them. As the validating caregiver, you move in closer. Touch can sometimes trigger feelings or memories for the person in Time Confusion or Repetitive Motion. When you are validating a person in Phase Four, Vegetation, touch is the most important technique to use. It is often the only way to make con-

Exercise: Linking Behavior with an Unmet Human Need

Purpose—To practice communicating by exploring an unmet human need

Very old people who are in Phases 2 and 3 and have lost dictionary words communicate their human needs through some kind of movement. The validating caregiver verbalizes their unmet human needs in order to build empathy and help them meet their needs for the moment.

Instructions

Pair up into dyads and face one another.

Instructor to "A": Say a word that is a noun that has meaning for you, like "mother," "book," "dog," "pillow" with emotion.

Instructor to "B": Try to identify the emotion expressed by "A" and match it to a basic human need [*use the overhead for reference*]. Then, give me a sentence that connects the emotion with the need. Here's some examples: "A" says "mother," you say, "You miss your mother." "A" says "book," you say, "You love to read."

Communicate like this for about 3 minutes, then switch roles.

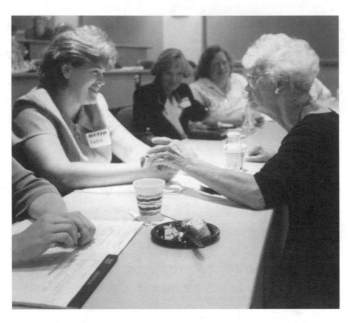

A demonstration of using touch in Validation.

tact. I'm going to distribute a handout that describes some ways of touching in Validation that Feil has found can bring about a strong response in people who are in Phases 2, 3, or 4.

> (Distribute the handout "Using Touch in Validation."
> Allow time for participants to read it.
> Conduct the exercise on touching in Validation.)

INSTRUCTOR:　Here's an exercise we can do to practice using the various ways of touching. Remember that as validating caregivers, we can become substitutes for loved ones. We can stimulate feelings or memories of "mother," "father," "sibling," "colleague," "partner/loved one," or "children."

Using Music

INSTRUCTOR:　The final Validation technique is music. Some therapists who work with very old people believe that our ability to comprehend music is the last thing to go before we die. The music that we've known and loved from our very earliest days stays with us throughout life. Very old people who have become nonverbal by reason of disuse or even stroke actually can still sing all of the words to familiar songs from the past and thoroughly enjoy it. Music is an invaluable tool that can be used in any phase of Resolution. The Validation practitioner must have a good repertoire of songs and the ability to pull them out at appropriate times, and if any-

Exercise: Using Touch in Validation

Purpose—To connect with very old people in Phases 2, 3, or 4 of Resolution and to communicate through touching

Instructions

Get into pairs and sit facing one another, close together so that you can touch. Choose who will be "A" and who will be "B." Take a breath and center.

Instructor to "A": Close your eyes, and think of your mother, father, or one of your siblings. Don't say anything, just create a visual image of this person using your mind's eye. Can you see this person's face? The chin? Eyes? Mouth? Shoulders? Typical posture? What does this person usually wear? Can you hear their voice? What are they saying? Is the voice high or low? Fast or slow? Does this person have a particular smell? What do you feel when you are near this person? Where do you feel that in your body? Keep your eyes closed.

Instructor to "B": OK, during all this, I want you to observe your partner carefully. Look for changes in the face, breathing, posture, way of holding hands, position of the feet—everything. Take it all in. Can you sense a change in their energy? Try to use your intuition and feel who your partner is thinking about. Use appropriate touch for that person.

Instructor to "A": If the touch matches who you're thinking about "A," open your eyes.

Instructor to "B": If it wasn't the right person, keep trying. Concentrate.

When "B" figures out who the person is, allow "A" and "B" to switch roles and lead the exercise again.

thing about a particular client's music preferences is known, so much the better. Maybe there's a song that can be tied to the person's experience—a job or geographic location, for instance. Music also can be a way of expressing feelings. You can find a song to match any mood. Sharing music of any kind together promotes trust, empathy, cooperation, and communication. Here's a list of songs that should be familiar to the people you're caring for.

(Distribute handout "Classic Songs."
Ask participants to add to the list.)

INSTRUCTOR: Often, a person in Vegetation will respond to some form of music, especially if the song is an old favorite or has personal meaning. Of course, music therapy is an art all its own, but as we use it in Validation, music is a simple, informal, and spontaneous means of communication that energizes and reduces anxiety in older people.

(If time permits, have a brief sing-along
using one of the songs on the "Classic Songs" list.
You also could conduct the exercise "Music and Mirroring.")

INSTRUCTOR: We're going to divide into pairs again. This time, each pair is going to work out a role play that will demonstrate some of the Validation techniques. I'll give each of you an assignment. You can use these examples, or you can make up an example or draw from your own experience and end up with something better. You can look at some of the stories in *The Validation Breakthrough* for ideas. The purpose here is to give a correct demonstration of the techniques.

(Allow about 30 minutes for preparation of the role plays.
Let each dyad present their assigned technique, with the group
offering a critique. If there is time, suggest that the "wrong way" as
well as the "right way" of demonstrating Validation. Display the
overhead transparency "Phases of Resolution and the Appropriate
Validation Techniques" as a quick review and summary. Allow 45
minutes to 1 hour for role plays and critique/discussion.)

Exercise: Music and Mirroring

Purpose—To practice mirroring movement with people in Phase 3 of Resolution

Many older people who have lost the ability to speak can still sing. They may not remember the name of the song, but when the validating caregiver begins to sing the words, the old person can sing the entire song.

Instructions

"A" and "B" stand and face one another. Each should take time to center.

"A" sings a familiar song, such as "You Are My Sunshine."

"B" watches "A's" lips and eyes and listens to "A's" pitch and tempo.

"B" mirrors "A's" lip movements and adjusts his or her pitch and tempo to "A's."

Feedback

Instructor to both: How did you feel doing this exercise? Do you feel closer to each other?

4 Putting It All Together

INSTRUCTOR: We have learned about and practiced individual Validation techniques. All that's left is putting it all together and applying the techniques in a Validation "session" or "moment." What exactly is a Validation session or moment? When is the best time to use Validation?

(Allow time for a few responses.)

INSTRUCTOR: You don't need to go into a special room or private place and talk to a very old disoriented person for 15 minutes or a half-hour. You don't need to have a special place or a time or set up. All you need is to be centered and open. You can practice Validation while you are doing some other activity, like helping someone get dressed or while bathing. A session or moment can last 3 minutes or 15 minutes depending on the person's concentration level and the amount of time you have. The most important thing to remember is to use common sense and work from your heart. If you go to a person with the intention of validating him or her, and that person doesn't feel like communicating, it's not going to work. The best time to validate someone is when the client wants to communicate and when you are centered, ready to be empathetic and open to that communication. I'm generalizing here. Can you think of specific times during a workday when it would be good to use Validation?

(Allow time for a few responses. Make sure the range of responses includes when a client is sitting in the day room, pacing the halls, pounding on doors, crying, eating meals, bathing, dressing, drinking coffee, and the practitioner has a free 5 minutes.)

INSTRUCTOR: Okay. Those times are all good. Let's summarize. You can validate someone anytime, including during the course of your normal activities. A Validation session or moment can last 3 minutes—the length of time it takes to sing a familiar song—or as long as 15–20 minutes, if the client feels like talking and you have the time.

Starting a Validation Session

INSTRUCTOR: Let's move on to putting together a Validation session. The first thing you need to do is center: Clear your mind of any inner thoughts or feelings that can get in the way of building empathy with your client. Concentrate on the person you're working with. The second step is to observe the person carefully. You practiced precise observation in Level 1 to assess the phase of Resolution the person was in, but let's do it again. Start at the top of the person's head and go down to the toes. What does he or she look like today? What feelings (if any) are being expressed? What basic human need (if any) is being expressed? Begin the process of building empathy by matching or mirroring what you see at a distance. Once you feel a connection with the person, physically move toward him or her. Move close enough for the disoriented person to know that you are there, but remember to be aware of the distance between you. If the person is still verbal, then you can introduce yourself. Use a handshake—it's a nice way to show respect for and make physical contact with someone who is Maloriented. Someone who is Time Confused may need more physical contact, touching, and eye contact. A person in Repetitive Motion needs to know that you are there—move in close; a pat on the hand or knee is not enough. Remember that damage to the kinesthetic sense, which senses feeling, comes with getting older. Also, the circulation is not as good, so a very old disoriented person may not even know that you are there if you are just patting the knee or hand. You need to get closer; move into their personal space. And, of course, working with someone in Vegetation requires touching and getting very close to him or her.

Start by asking nonthreatening, factual questions of people who are in Phase 1 and 2, using mirroring with someone in Phase 3, and touching techniques with someone in Phase 4. These certainly are not hard-and-fast rules but simple hints as to how to begin. It's often difficult in the beginning to know what to ask or which technique to use when. With practice, you'll stop thinking about it and simply relate to the person, verbally or nonverbally, or both. When you do, you'll know that you have integrated the techniques and the principles of Validation.

Ending a Validation Session

INSTRUCTOR: Ending a Validation session with a very old disoriented or confused person appropriately is extremely important. Whether the person is Maloriented or disoriented, you have a relationship with that person, which you've established through your words, eye contact, touch, and empathy. You can't walk away and say, "Well, goodbye. See you later. Nice talking to you." You have to give the person some acknowledgment that you value the relationship and the conversations you've had. Let them know that you do have to go now, but you will be back. It's not just a casual hello–goodbye thing. You can take the person's hand and look into his or her eyes and say with real sincerity in your voice, "I have to go now, Mrs. Cohn, but I'll be back tomorrow afternoon at about the same time," and make very sure that you are. If you don't return, you'll destroy the trust you've built between you, and that trust is essential to validating someone successfully.

(Ask participants to suggest other ways to end a session appropriately, or tell the class the things that have worked for them. Allow a few minutes for responses.)

INSTRUCTOR: Let's put it all together using role play. Break up into groups of two. Each of you will have a chance to role play a very old disoriented person and a Validation caregiver. Don't be nervous—remember, this is not an acting class. Take a few minutes to choose a disoriented older adult either from your work experience or from *The Validation Breakthrough*. The other person will use whatever techniques are necessary to make contact with the person and conduct a brief Validation session. Decide who will be "A," a very old disoriented person, and who will be "B," the validator. Take a moment to center. I'm going to help the person who is role-playing the client.

Instructor to "A": What does this very old person look like? What does his or her hair look like? Can you see his or her face? Are the lips tight or hanging loose? See the shoulders? Are they slumped over or straight? Is the breathing fast or slow? Shallow or deep? What clothes is this person wearing? How does this person walk or move? Can you see this person's hands? What does this person sound like? Can you hear his or her voice? Does he speak or make sounds? Is the voice high or low? Does she speak quickly or slowly? Now, "become" that person.

Instructor to "B": Observe "A" carefully. When you are ready, move toward "A" and initiate a brief Validation session.

(Allow no more than 10 minutes for this role play.)

Instructor to "B": Give "A" feedback on which techniques worked for you and which did not.

Switch roles and repeat the exercise role-play.

Note: You can spend as much time as you want role-playing. Role-play in front of the entire group so that everyone can give feedback. An effective teaching method is for you to role-play with various students: You play the validating caregiver while students role-play very old disoriented people. This teaching tool helps you to demonstrate "the right way" to validate.

Summary

INSTRUCTOR: We've come to the end of the training. I hope that you have learned practical ways of communicating and helping very old disoriented people and that you feel ready to go out and practice what we've learned together. You now have the building blocks that you need to use Validation. You won't do it all perfectly in the beginning, but trust that it's okay to make mistakes. The very old disoriented person will forgive you for making mistakes because he or she knows that you are honest and you care. Keep on trying! When you have doubts, refer to your copy of *The Validation Breakthrough* and review the principles of Validation. You know you can always turn to empathizing, caring, and building a trusting relationship. Everything else is just icing on the cake!

I would like to encourage anyone who wants to go further with Validation to work toward certification. There are three levels of certification: a certified Validation worker, a certified Validation group leader, and a certified Validation teacher/ trainer. A certified Validation worker is trained to demonstrate individual Validation and show colleagues how to practice it. A certified Validation group leader is trained to do group Validation to show colleagues how to practice it. A certified teacher/ trainer can teach Validation. If you are interested, please see me.

Thank you for all your hard work. Good luck and have fun!

Study Guide for *The Four Phases of Resolution*

Pose the following questions to the group to answer after viewing the video:

1. What is meant by the sentence "There is meaning behind the behavior of very old disoriented people?"
2. How is this sentence illustrated in the video?
3. What is the meaning behind the hoarding behavior of the Maloriented old woman? What is meant when she accuses her caregiver of poisoning her food?
4. The Maloriented woman is incontinent, but she cannot admit it. How does that explain her refusal to take a bath?
5. Why can't the Time Confused old woman recognize her caregiver?
6. What unresolved issue did the Time Confused woman face when she searched for her father?
7. How do you explain the final Resolution struggle for very old disoriented people?
8. Why does the person in Repetitive Motion use human body parts to express human needs?
9. What are the physical characteristics of a person in Vegetation?
10. What are the basic human needs of very old people in the final Resolution struggle?
11. What emotions do they express?

Study Guide
for *100 Years to Live*

Pose the following questions to the group to answer after viewing the video:

1. Why did the daughters have trouble getting social services for their aged mothers?
2. Was the move to a nursing facility appropriate?
3. Is the government responsible for providing social services to all older adults?
4. What responsibility do adult children, grandchildren, and great-grandchildren have for their older adult family members?
5. Is living together always the best way for several generations of family?
6. What life task did Mrs. Dorsey not face successfully?
7. When Mrs. Dorsey lost her role, she said, "You lose everything to your name . . . you're driving me crazy." Does losing one's lifetime role mean losing one's adult controls?
8. Can we prepare for the losses associated with aging? How?
9. Why do strong emotions sometimes build up during a lifetime and spill over in old age?
10. Can we learn to face each small "death" during each life stage?
11. Should healthy aging be taught in school? At what age?
12. Does acknowledging a loss help to relieve it?
13. The social worker remained detached in her initial interviews with Mrs. Dorsey and Mrs. Aiken. Was this approach helpful or was it detrimental?
14. When is sympathetic intimacy helpful? When do very old people need warm nurturing?
15. Mrs. Aiken's house was sold. Was the broken furnace a ploy used by the family to avoid telling her the painful truth? Is it ever wise to lie to very old people?
16. Did Mrs. Dorsey recreate her past in fantasy form to forget the painful present reality? Did she choose to remember pleasurable past experiences?

17. In the city hospital Mrs. Dorsey said, "I didn't know it was so late." Was she speaking of her life time rather than the clock time?

18. Mrs. Dorsey longed to live. Was that wise?

19. Mrs. Aiken kept her sense of humor and her ability to relate to people in present time. Have you experienced a situation in which a sense of humor helped you overcome a loss?

Study Guide for
The Seminar Group

Pose the following questions to the group to answer after viewing the video:

1. What methods for aging successfully do the members of the seminar group have in common?
2. What do you think is the most important quality needed for successful aging?
3. How did these very old people view the future?
4. Were the people in this video able to compromise at the end of life?
5. Did the 94-year-old woman have integrity?
6. How would you define *integrity*?

The Validation Training Program. ©1999 Naomi Feil. All rights reserved.

Phases of Resolution and Their Appropriate Validation Techniques

Phase One
Malorientation

Centering
Asking factual
    questions
Rephrasing
Identifying and
    using the
    preferred sense
Asking the
    extreme
Imagining the
    opposite
Reminiscing

Phase Two
Time Confusion

Centering
Touching
Maintaining eye contact
    and a caring tone of
    voice
Observing, matching
    and expressing the
    emotion with
    emotion
Using ambiguity
Linking behavior with a
    basic human need
Using music

Phase Three
Repetitive Motion

Centering
Touching
Linking behavior
    with a basic
    human need
Using music
Mirroring

Phase Four
Vegetation

Centering
Using music
Using sensory
    stimulation
Touching

Keep in mind that many techniques are used in several phases of Resolution. Just because a technique is listed under a particular phase does not mean that it cannot be used with other phases; each technique is associated with the phase where it is used the most. Verbal techniques such as asking factual questions, asking the extreme, imagining the opposite, and reminiscing, also can be used to a large extent with Time Confused individuals. Observing, matching, and expressing the emotion also are appropriate for very old people in Repetitive Motion.

The most important factor to remember is that there is no prescription; each person is unique and will respond in his or her individual way. It is more important for the Validation caregiver to respond to the very old disoriented person with respect and empathy. Even if you make a mistake, the person will forgive you as long as you have used empathy, caring, and respect in dealing with him or her.

The Validation Training Program. ©1999 Naomi Feil. All rights reserved.

Words that Relate to a Person's Preferred Sense

Auditory	Kinesthetic	Visual
Tune	Touch	Picture
Note	Handle	Clear
Accent	Throw	Focus
Ring	Finger	Perspective
Shout	Shock	See
Growl	Stir	Flash
Tone	Strike	Bright
Sing	Impress	Outlook
Sound	Move	Spectacle
Hear	Hit	Glimpse
Clear	Grope	Preview
Say	Impact	Shortsighted
Scream	Stroke	Discern
Click	Tap	Distinguish
Static	Rub	Illustrate
Rattle	Crash	Delineate
Ask	Smash	Paint
Chord	Sharpen	Cloud
Amplify	Tangible	Clarify
Harmonize	Crawl	Graphic
Key	Irritate	Dress up
Muffle	Tickle	Show
Voice	Sore	Reveal
Compose	Grab	Expose
Alarm	Carry	Depict
Screech	Flat	Screen

Using Touch in Validation

Touching clients is an effective nonverbal communication technique. Touching another human being is an act of intimacy, and caregivers, both professional and family, always must respect that some people, even when their controls are damaged, may not want to be touched. Any sign of resistance to physical contact should indicate to the caregiver that touching is not appropriate. The personal space of all people, whether they are disoriented or not, always must be respected.

Where you touch the person is important. Because early, emotionally tinged memories are permanently imprinted in the circuitry of the brain, the Validation caregiver can kindle a significant relationship by touching people in Repetitive Motion in the same way that they were touched by a loved one in childhood. The following are special touching techniques that may be effective when used with people who are in Stages 2 or 3; people in Stage 1 are rarely receptive to touch.

- Using the palm of the hand, touch the upper cheek in a light, circular motion. This stimulates feelings of "being mothered," memories of the relationship with mother. Using the hand in this way is a familiar "rooting" reflex.

- Using the fingertips on the back of the head, move in a circular motion with a moderate amount of pressure. This stimulates feelings of "being fathered," memories of the relationship with father, being patted on the head as a child.

- Using the outside of the hand, place the little finger under the earlobe and curve along the chin with both hands in a soft, stroking motion downward along the jaw. This stimulates memories of having a spouse or lover.

- Using both hands, cup the fingers on the back of the neck and stroke in a small, circular motion. This stimulates memories of mother or father touching the person as a child.

- Using the full hand, rub with full pressure the shoulders or upper back near the shoulder blades. This stimulates memories of being a sibling or good friend, or a relationship with a brother or sister.

- Touching the inside of the calf near the knee with the fingertips stimulates memories of caring for animals, such as horses and cows.

Classic Songs

Amazing Grace
America (My Country, 'Tis of Thee)
America the Beautiful
Battle Hymn of the Republic
Blue Skies
Daisy, Daisy
Danny Boy
De Colores
Dona Nobis Pacem
Do-Re-Mi
Down by the Riverside
Frere Jacques
Give My Regards to Broadway
God Bless America
The Green, Green Grass of Home
Havah Nagilah
He's Got the Whole World in His Hands
Home on the Range
I've Been Working on the Railroad
I Want a Girl
If I Had a Hammer
It's a Long Way to Tipperary

Jesus Loves Me
Jingle Bells
Let Me Call You Sweetheart
Let There Be Peace on Earth
Lift Ev'ry Voice and Sing
Michael (Row the Boat Ashore)
The More We Get Together
Music Alone Shall Live
My Bonnie Lies Over the Ocean
Oh! Susanna
Over My Head
Rock-A-My Soul
Shalom Chaverim
She'll Be Comin' 'Round the Mountain
Shenandoah
Simple Gifts
Sometimes I Feel Like a Motherless Child
The Star-Spangled Banner
Swing Low, Sweet Chariot
This Land Is Your Land
This Little Light of Mine
You Are My Sunshine
You Take the High Road
When Irish Eyes Are Smiling

Bibliography

Aiken, L. (1995). *Aging: An introduction to gerontology.* Thousand Oaks, CA: Sage Publications.

Alzheimer, A. (1907). Über eine eigenartige Erkrankung der Hirnrinds. *Allgemeine Zeitschrift für Psychiatrie, 64,* 146–148.

Arking, R. (1998). *Biology of aging* (2nd ed., pp. 155–162). Sunderland, MA: Sinauer Associates.

Atchley, R.C. (1991). *Social forces and aging* (6th ed.). Belmont, CA: Wadsworth.

Billig, N. (1993). *Growing older and wiser.* New York: Lexington Books.

Birren, J.E. (Ed.). (1996). *Encyclopedia of gerontology: Aging and the aged.* San Diego: Academic Press.

Birren, J.E., & Schaie, J.W. (1996). *Handbook of the psychology of aging* (4th ed.). San Diego: Academic Press.

Butler, R.N. (1963). The life review: An interpretation of reminiscence in the aged. *Psychiatry, 26,* 65–75.

Butler, R.N., & Lewis, M. (1977). *Aging and mental health.* St. Louis: Mosby.

Dietch, J.T., Hewett, L.J., & Jones, S. (1989). Adverse effects of reality orientation. *Journal of the American Geriatrics Society, 37,* 974–976.

Erikson, E. (1963). *Childhood and society.* New York: W.W. Norton.

Feil, N. (1985). RESOLUTION: The final life task. *Journal of Humanistic Psychology, 25,* 91–105.

Feil, N. (1989). Validation®: An empathetic approach to the care of dementia. *Clinical Gerontologist, 8,* 89–94.

Feil, N. (1991). Validation® therapy. In P.K.H. Kim (Ed.), *Serving the elderly* (pp. 89–114). New York: Aldine de Gruyter.

Feil, N. (1992a). Validation® therapy with late onset dementia populations. In G. Jones & B.M.L. Miesen (Eds.), *Caregiving in dementia* (pp. 199–218). London: Routledge.

Feil, N. (1992b). *V/F Validation: The Feil method* (rev. ed.). Cleveland: Feil Productions.

Feil, N., & Flynn, J. (1983). Meaning behind movements of the disoriented old-old. *Somatics, 4,* 4–10.

Freud, S. (1938). *Basic writings of Sigmund Freud,* Vol. 1: *The psychopathology of everyday life.* New York: Random House.

Fritz, P. (1986). *The language of RESOLUTION among the old-old: The effect of validation therapy on two levels of cognitive confusion.* Research results presented to the Speech Communication Association, Chicago.

Hayslip, B., Jr., & Panek, P.E. (1989). *Adult development and aging.* New York: Harper & Row.

Hendricks, T., & Wills, R. (1975). *The centering book.* Upper Saddle River, NJ: Prentice Hall.

Maddox, G. (1995). *The encyclopedia of aging* (2nd ed.). New York: Springer.

Papalio, D.E., Camp, J., & Feldman, R.D. (1996). *Adult development and aging.* New York: McGraw-Hill.

Penfield, W. (1975). *The mystery of the mind* (pp. 21–36). Princeton, NJ: Princeton University Press.

Piaget, J. (1952). *The origins of intelligence in children.* New York: W.W. Norton.

Pipher, M. (1999). *Another country: Navigating the emotional terrain of our elders.* New York: Penguin.

Rogers, C. (1981). *A way of being.* Boston: Houghton Mifflin.

Ordering Information

Books

The Validation Breakthrough: Simple Techniques for Communicating with People with "Alzheimer's-Type Dementia," by Naomi Feil, ©1993, $22.95
Order from Health Professions Press, P.O. Box 10624, Baltimore, MD 21285-0624. Specify Stock Number 0114. Phone (888) 337-8808, Fax (410) 337-8539, www.healthpropress.com.

Validation: The Feil Method, by Naomi Feil, revised 1992
Order from Edward Feil Productions, 4614 Prospect Avenue, Cleveland, OH 44103. Phone (216) 881-0040, Fax (216) 751-6434.

Videos

Communicating with the Alzheimer's-Type Population (19 minutes)
Validation techniques are demonstrated clearly in before-and-after role-plays. ($99.00) (Also available from Health Professions Press)

Looking for Yesterday (29 minutes)
The development of Validation with very old disoriented nursing facility residents is documented. ($99.00)

The More We Get Together (44 minutes)
Part One clearly explains the phases of Resolution by documenting people in each phase. Part Two documents a Validation group session. ($150)

These videos can be rented (fee information available) or purchased through Edward Feil Productions.

The Validation® Training Program
Boxed set of 2 training manuals, 2 VHS videocassettes, set of 21 overheads at $355.00 (individual components total $395.00). Specify Stock Number 2564. All components © 1999. Available from Health Professions Press.

Individual Components
  Validation Training Manual, Level 1, Stock Number 2513, 112 pages, $28.00.
  Validation Training Manual, Level 2, Stock Number 2521, 80 pages, $24.00.
  Validation Training Video: *Coping,* Stock Number 253X, 40-minute VHS, $175.00.
  Validation Training Video: *Resolution,* Stock Number 2548, 30-minute VHS, $150.00.
  Overhead transparencies, Stock Number 2556, 21 acetate sheets with folder, $25.00.

Prices are subject to change without notice and may be higher outside the United States.